NATURAL POWER

CURE FOR DISEASES

ABHIJIT DAS

NATURAL
CURE FOR DISEASES
POWER

"Natural Power: Cure for Diseases" is a book that presents the latest approaches in the field of health and treatment. This book offers solutions for diseases using various natural elements and techniques, enriching physical, mental, and spiritual health. It presents solutions for diseases through different natural remedies and techniques, providing guidance towards a balanced and healthy life.

ABHIJIT DAS

E-Book Price : Rs. 399.00 Only.
Copyright © 2024 Abhijit Das
Contact: +91 98644 96332

Disclaimer

"Please note: This book is intended for educational and informational purposes only and should not be taken as any kind of medical or therapeutic advice. Consult an expert or physician before addressing any medical problem. The main purpose of our book is to spread education and awareness. We recommend purchasing it because it includes information about medicine, Ayurveda, and natural treatments that can help you towards better health and life. However, it is essential that everyone exercises caution and consults a professional physician before use. Every possible effort has been made to ensure the accuracy of the content; however, the author will not be responsible for any unintended errors. If any errors are found, corrective steps will be taken."

BEGINNING

There is a deep connection between the natural environment and human life. There are many ways to improve your self-confidence. Plants are one of nature's various contributions that have greatly impacted all of us. In this natural environment, there are many medicinal plants essential for our human life. There are also some essential medicinal plants around my house. A regional study of these essential medicinal plants should be conducted to prepare home-based remedies. This will help us learn about the properties and uses of the medicinal plants in the vicinity. After a regional study and an in-depth understanding of these medicinal plants, some households can prepare their own medicines and prevent various illnesses.

PURPOSE OF FIELD STUDY

The main objective of this project is to study various plants and generate knowledge. This study will help us examine natural conditions, allowing us to understand its natural balance. Additionally, through this study, we will attempt to identify medicinal plants, reliably understand their medicinal properties, and enhance the ability to use them for various ailments. This project is not only scientifically significant but also provides people with a new and natural remedy for improving health.

IT TOOK ME ABOUT 6 MONTHS TO COMPLETE THIS PROJECT.

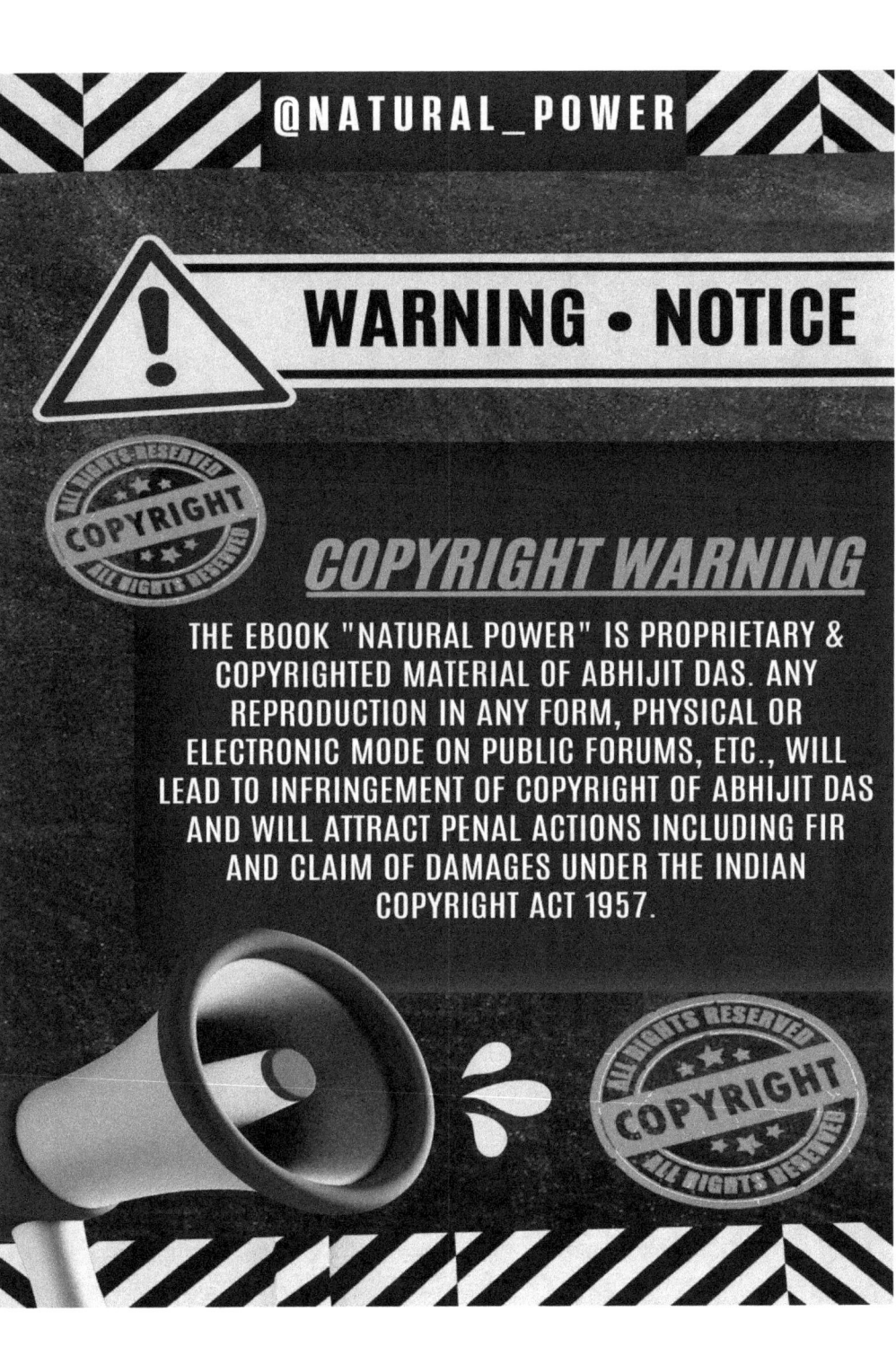

NATURAL POWER · CURE FOR DISEASES · ABHIJIT DAS

TABLE OF CONTENTS

- TULSI
- CURRY LEAVES
- NEEM
- INDIAN GOOSEBERRY
- CLOVE
- GUAVA
- TURMERIC
- BRAHMI
- MINT
- ASHWAGANDHA
- ALOE VERA
- GINGER
- LEMON
- FENUGREEK
- AJWAIN

NATURAL REMEDIES IN HEALTH PROTECTION: SOLUTIONS TO DISEASES

NATURAL POWER · CURE FOR DISEASES · ABHIJIT DAS

SCIENTIFIC NAME

- TULSI : OCIMUM TENUIFLORUM
- CURRY LEAVES : MURRAYA KOENIGII
- NEEM : AZADIRACHTA INDICA
- INDIAN GOOSEBERRY : PHYLLANTHUS EMBLICA
- CLOVE : SYZYGIUM AROMATICUM
- GUAVA : PSIDIUM GUAJAVA
- TURMERIC : CURCUMA LONGA
- BRAHMI : BACOPA MONNIERI
- MINT : MENTHA
- ASHWAGANDHA : WITHANIA SOMNIFERA
- ALOE VERA : ALOE BARBADENSIS MILLER
- GINGER : ZINGIBER OFFICINALE
- LEMON : CITRUS LIMON
- FENUGREEK : TRIGONELLA FOENUM-GRAECUM
- AJWAIN : TRACHYSPERMUM AMMI

NATURAL REMEDIES IN HEALTH PROTECTION: SOLUTIONS TO DISEASES

1. <u>TULSI</u>:-

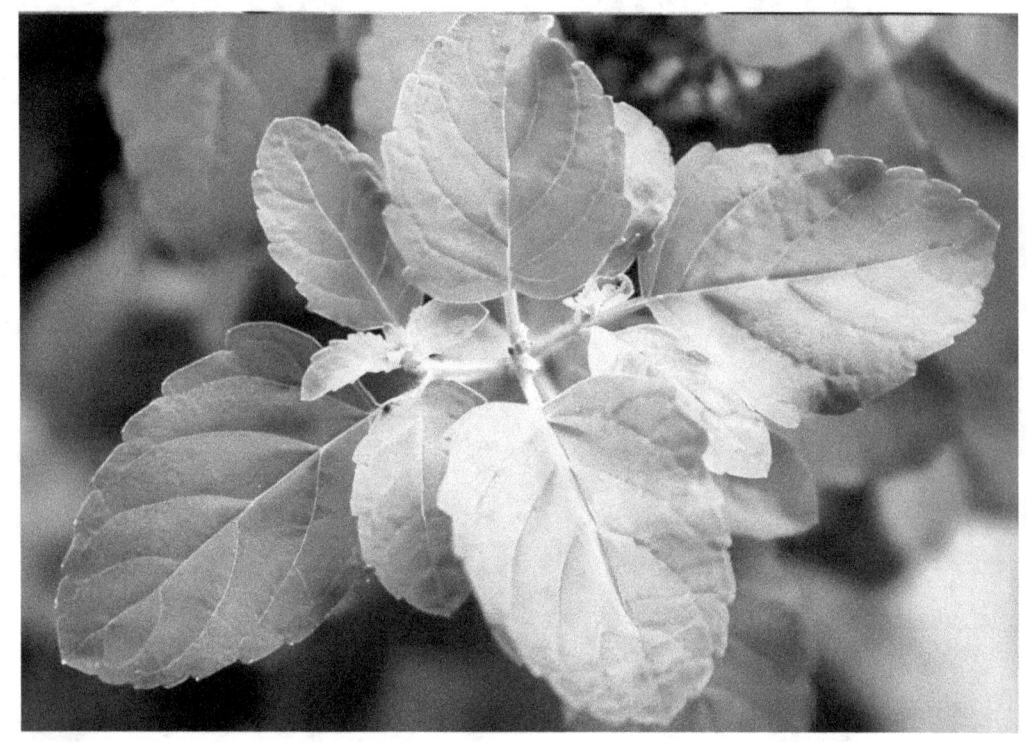

<u>Medicinal properties and uses</u>:-

The holy basil plant is endowed with medicinal properties. The leaves of holy basil are used to purify the blood. The tea made from holy basil leaves is used to treat liver diseases. Consuming holy basil juice helps in relieving nausea and cough. Additionally, regular consumption enhances skin complexion, improves overall body beauty, and reduces diabetes. Holy basil juice acts as an antiseptic for hair. Drinking a mixture of holy basil leaf juice and turmeric juice is better for high blood pressure. Mixing black salt and black pepper with black basil and drinking it relieves the hiccups. Besides worship, there are also many properties of basil leaves. If cough persists, drinking basil leaves and ginger mixed with honey is beneficial. Applying basil leaves to wounds helps to heal the wounds. Applying basil juice with coconut oil reduces the burning sensation in any part of the body. The burnt area dries quickly, and there are no stains. To improve memory and memory, basil leaves should be eaten daily. Eating basil leaves with tea can lead to a healthy life for a long time. Basil is also popular as tea in many places. Basil enhances the immune system's resistance. Basil is used to make toothpaste because it is beneficial in dental diseases.

2. <u>CURRY LEAVES</u>:-

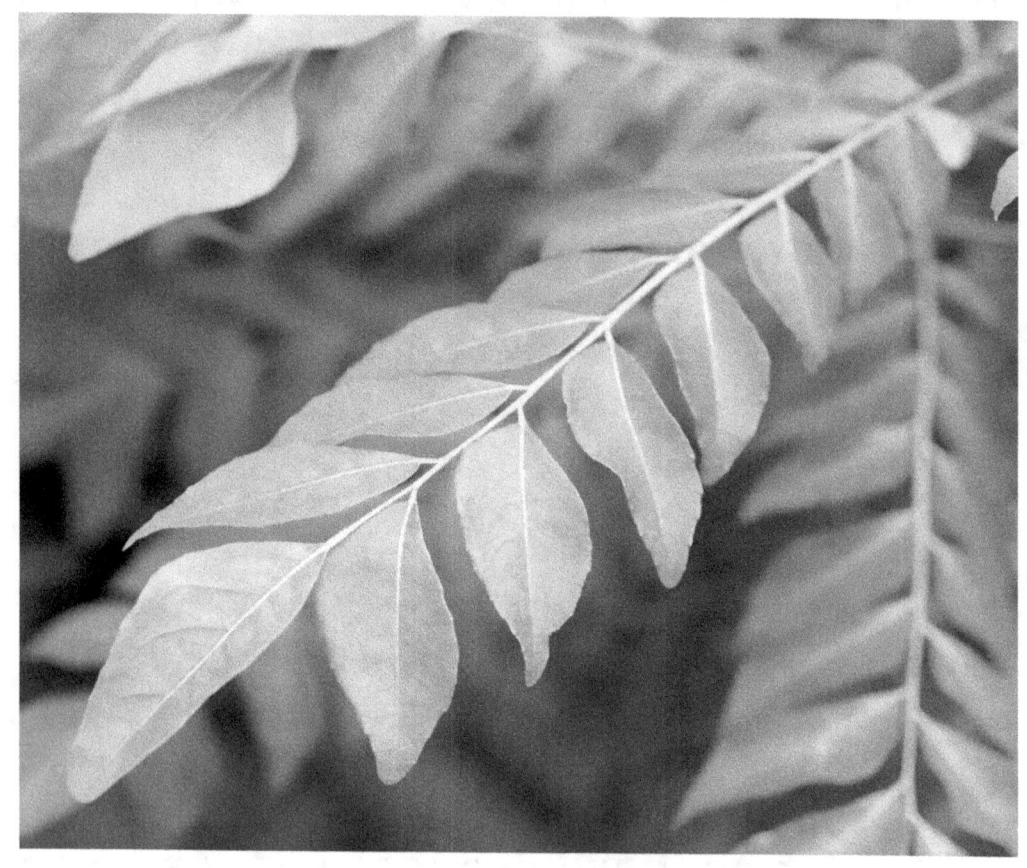

<u>Medicinal properties and uses</u>:-

This leaf is beneficial for children because it contains ample amounts of minerals, Vitamin A, Vitamin B, Vitamin C, and Vitamin E.

The medicinal properties and uses of curry leaves are listed below:-

Curry leaves enhance the beauty of hair and nails. Eating curry leaves can benefit pregnant women. Curry leaves contain a significant amount of iron, so consuming them increases blood in the body. Applying curry leaves to burnt areas provides relief from burns. The juice of these leaves increases the amount of blood in the body. Use the leaves of the curry tree if there is itching in the body. If there is pain in the stomach, it is better to take the juice of its leaves with the juice of ginger. If an insect or poisonous animal bites, it is better to repeatedly apply lemon juice mixed with the same amount of curry leaves juice to the injured area.

3. <u>NEEM</u>:-

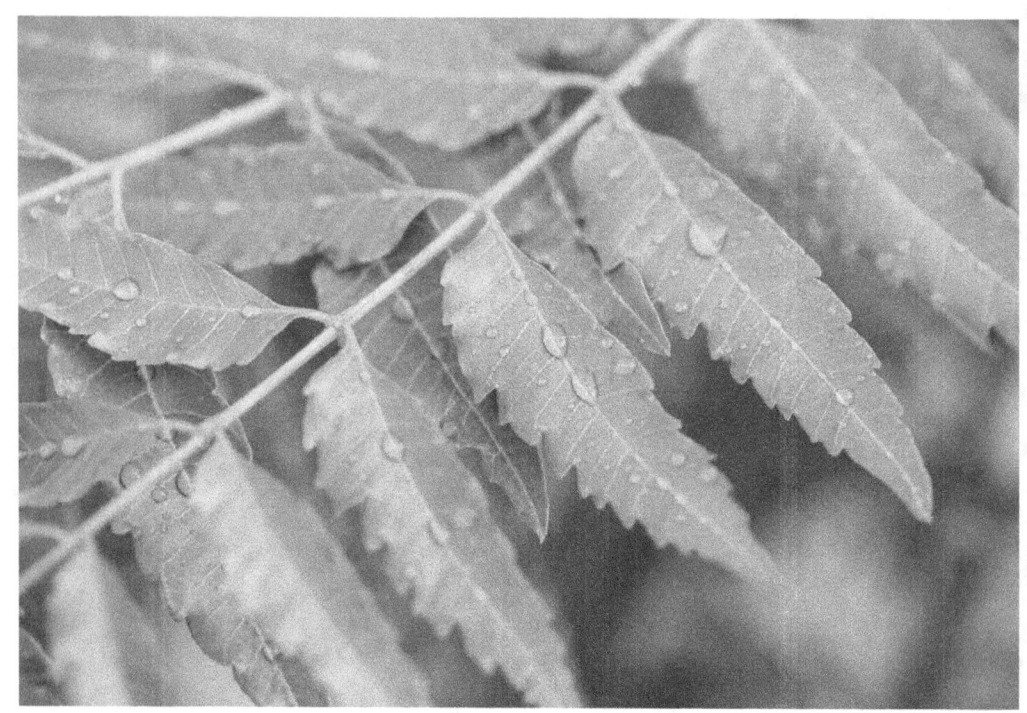

<u>Medicinal properties and uses</u>:-

Neem, a significant tree found in India, Pakistan, and Bangladesh, grows rapidly and is easily identifiable. It can reach heights of approximately 15-20 meters, with broad and drooping branches. Neem flowers are white and fragrant in nature, while its fruits are yellowish-white in color. In India, neem is revered as a sacred tree and is also used as a pharmacy in villages. Products made from the neem tree and the use of neem leaves are employed in the treatment of various diseases. Neem leaves are used to treat skin and gastrointestinal ailments. Additionally, neem leaves possess numerous medicinal properties beneficial for health. Each part of the neem tree has remarkable characteristics and is used in various treatments due to its excellent antibacterial, antifungal, and antiviral properties. Neem is an excellent remedy for hair and also beneficial for skin protection. Furthermore, neem leaf juice is used as a natural dietary supplement. Experiencing neem is extremely important as it can assist in protecting health and the environment.

4. <u>INDIAN GOOSEBERRY</u>:-

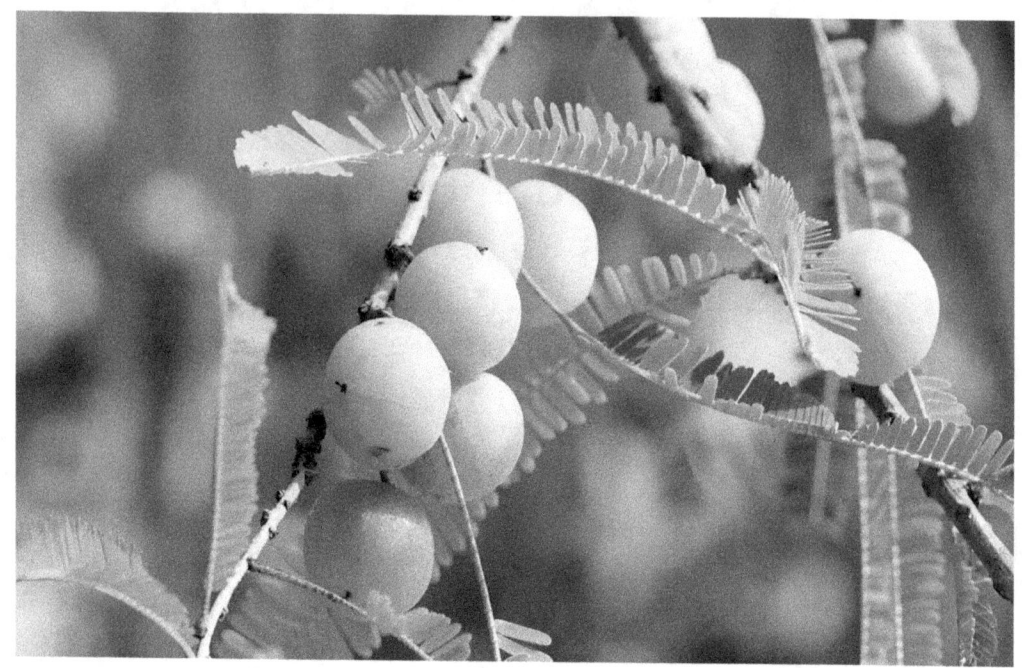

<u>Medicinal properties and uses</u>:-

Amla is a fruit that not only provides us with health benefits but also offers a delightful taste experience. It is a good source of Vitamin C, which enhances our immune system and protects the body from various infections. For diabetic patients, amla is extremely beneficial. Along with other elements, it helps in controlling blood sugar levels and managing their condition. Consumption of amla also alleviates acidity and gas problems. Additionally, when taken with honey, its benefits are further enhanced. Amla is beneficial for teeth, skin, and hair as well. It contains Vitamin C and calcium, which strengthen our body, ensuring the health of our skin, hair, and teeth. Therefore, amla not only maintains our physical health but also provides us with delicious and nutritious food. So, include amla in your diet today and keep yourself healthy.

5. <u>CLOVE</u>:-

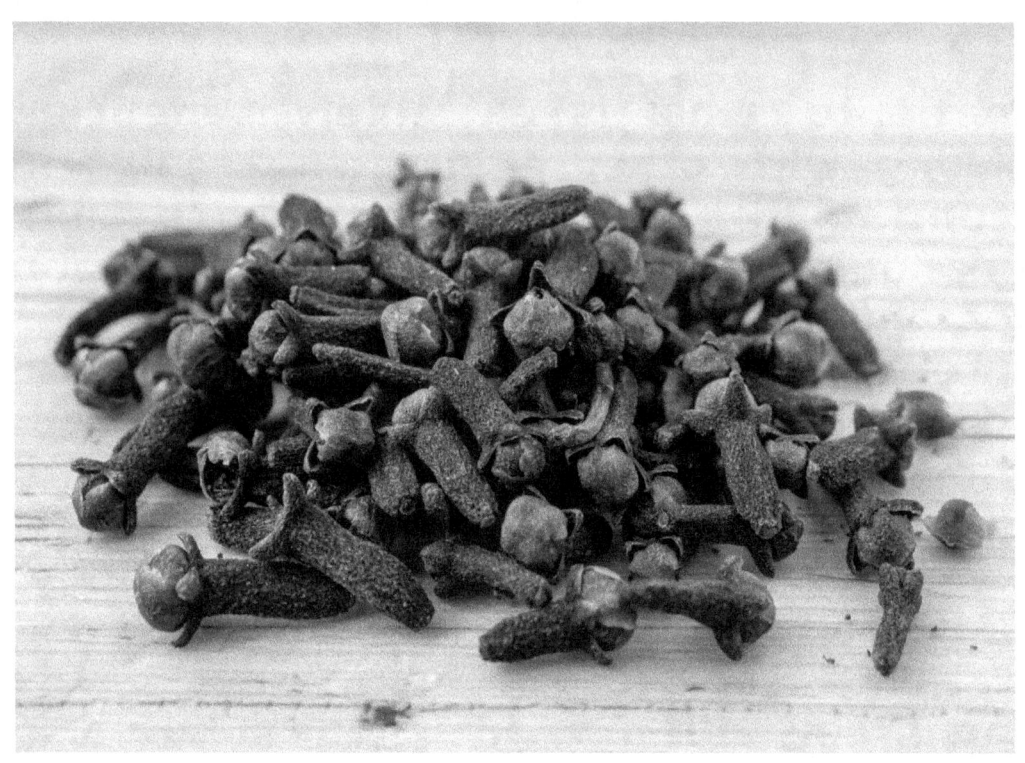

<u>Medicinal properties and uses</u>:-

Clove is a spice that not only makes your food delicious but also has medicinal properties that are beneficial for your health. Here are some medicinal benefits:

The antibacterial properties of clove can help reduce toothache.

I. Cloves can help eliminate bad breath.

II. Gargling with clove-infused warm water can relieve throat pain.

III. Consuming cloves or drinking clove-infused warm water can relieve cough.

IV. Consuming cloves can help relieve stomach gas.

V. Cloves can benefit people who suffer from persistent hiccups.

VI. Cloves enhance appetite and digestion, helping to prevent difficulties.

VII. Cloves can be beneficial for people suffering from tuberculosis.

Clove is a powerful and Ayurvedic spice that not only makes our food tasty but also provides health benefits due to its medicinal properties. The above benefits make it clear that regular consumption of cloves is important for a balanced and healthy lifestyle.

6. <u>GUAVA</u>:-

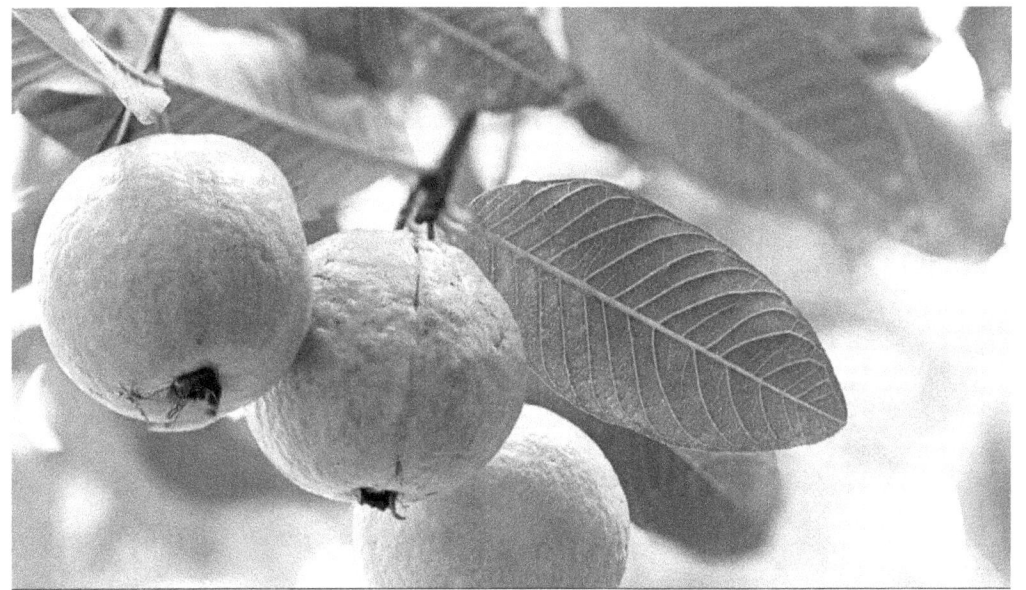

<u>Medicinal properties and uses</u>:-

Guava, which is called "Amrood" in Hindi, is a popular and delicious fruit grown in tropical and subtropical regions. This plant is rich in nutrients, and its fruits, leaves, and bark all have medicinal importance. Consuming guava is not only tasty but also extremely beneficial for health.

Medicinal properties:-

1. Rich in Vitamins and Minerals:- Guava is abundant in vitamins C, A, E, and B complex, as well as potassium, magnesium, and phosphorus. The amount of vitamin C in guava is four times higher than that in oranges, which strengthens the immune system.

2. Antioxidant Properties:- The antioxidants present in guava, such as carotene and lycopene, help fight free radicals in the body and protect cells from damage.

3. Improves Digestion:- Guava is high in fiber, which keeps the digestive system healthy and helps relieve constipation.

4. Blood Sugar Control:- Consuming guava leaves helps regulate blood sugar levels, benefiting individuals with diabetes.

5. Heart Health:- Consuming guava is also beneficial for the heart as it helps control blood pressure and reduces cholesterol levels.

6. Beneficial for Skin:- Consuming guava and applying a paste of its leaves helps reduce skin problems like acne and wrinkles.

USES:-

1. Consumed as a Fruit:- Fresh guava can be eaten directly as a fruit. It can also be added to salads, made into juice, or blended into smoothies.

2. **Use of Leaves:-** Guava leaves can be brewed into tea, which helps with digestion and blood sugar control. A paste of the leaves can be applied to the skin.

3. **Decoction of Bark and Leaves:-** A decoction made from guava bark and leaves can be consumed to relieve diarrhea and other stomach disorders.

4. **Guava Juice:-** Guava juice is a good source of vitamin C and other nutrients. Drinking it regularly strengthens the immune system.

5. **Guava Oil:-** Oil extracted from guava seeds is beneficial for the skin and hair.

CONCLUSION:-

Guava is a versatile fruit that is extremely beneficial for health. Its fruit, leaves, and bark all possess medicinal properties that help in curing various ailments and maintaining overall body health. Regular consumption of guava not only improves digestion and the immune system but also benefits heart and skin health. Guava can be consumed and used in various forms, making it an important and useful herb.

7. TURMERIC:-

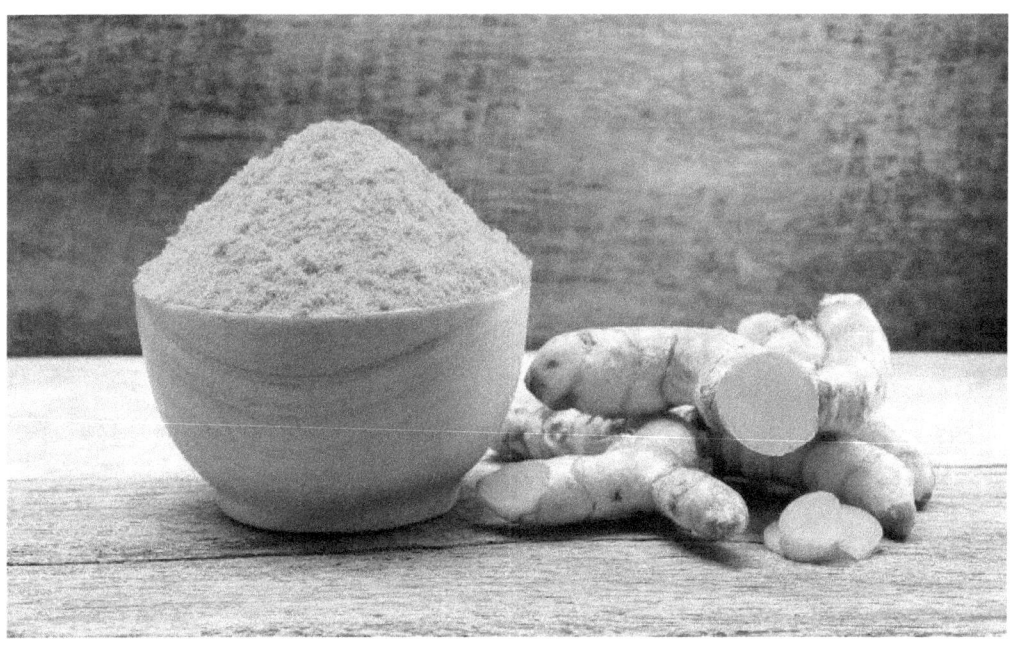

Medicinal properties and uses:-

Turmeric is a key spice widely used in Indian cuisine. Due to its medicinal properties, it also holds significant importance in Ayurvedic, Unani, and Chinese medical systems. The active ingredient in turmeric is 'curcumin,' which is considered responsible for many of its health benefits.

Medicinal properties:-

1. Anti-inflammatory properties:- Curcumin helps reduce inflammation. This property is useful in treating joint pain, arthritis, and other inflammation-related issues.

2. Antioxidant properties:- The curcumin present in turmeric is a powerful antioxidant that reduces free radicals in the body and protects against oxidative stress. It helps protect cells from damage.

3. Anti-bacterial and anti-viral properties:- Turmeric has natural anti-bacterial and anti-viral properties, which help in fighting infections and diseases.

4. Anti-cancer properties:- According to research, curcumin can help inhibit the growth of cancer cells and destroy them. It is particularly effective in colon, breast, and prostate cancers.

5. Digestive improvement:- Turmeric improves digestion and helps reduce stomach problems such as indigestion, gas, and bloating.

6. Beneficial for heart health:- Turmeric slows down the process of blood clotting, reducing the risk of heart attacks and strokes. It also helps in controlling cholesterol and blood pressure.

7. Beneficial for skin:- The antiseptic and anti-bacterial properties of turmeric help in treating skin problems such as acne, eczema, and psoriasis. It also helps in keeping the skin glowing and healthy.

USES:-

1. In food:- Turmeric is widely used in Indian cuisine. It is a key ingredient in vegetables, lentils, and spicy dishes.

2. With milk:- 'Turmeric milk' or 'golden milk' is a well-known home remedy useful in treating colds, coughs, and strengthening the immune system.

3. In skin treatments:- Turmeric is used in face masks, scrubs, and other skincare products.

4. As tea:- Turmeric tea is also popular and helps detoxify the body and reduce inflammation.

5. In Ayurvedic medicines:- Turmeric is used in various Ayurvedic medicines, which help in treating different diseases and disorders.

CONCLUSION:-

Turmeric is a versatile medicinal plant that has been used since ancient times for health improvement. Its anti-inflammatory, antioxidant, and anti-bacterial properties make it a unique natural remedy. Regular consumption of turmeric not only enhances the flavor of food but also provides numerous health benefits.

8. BRAHMI:-

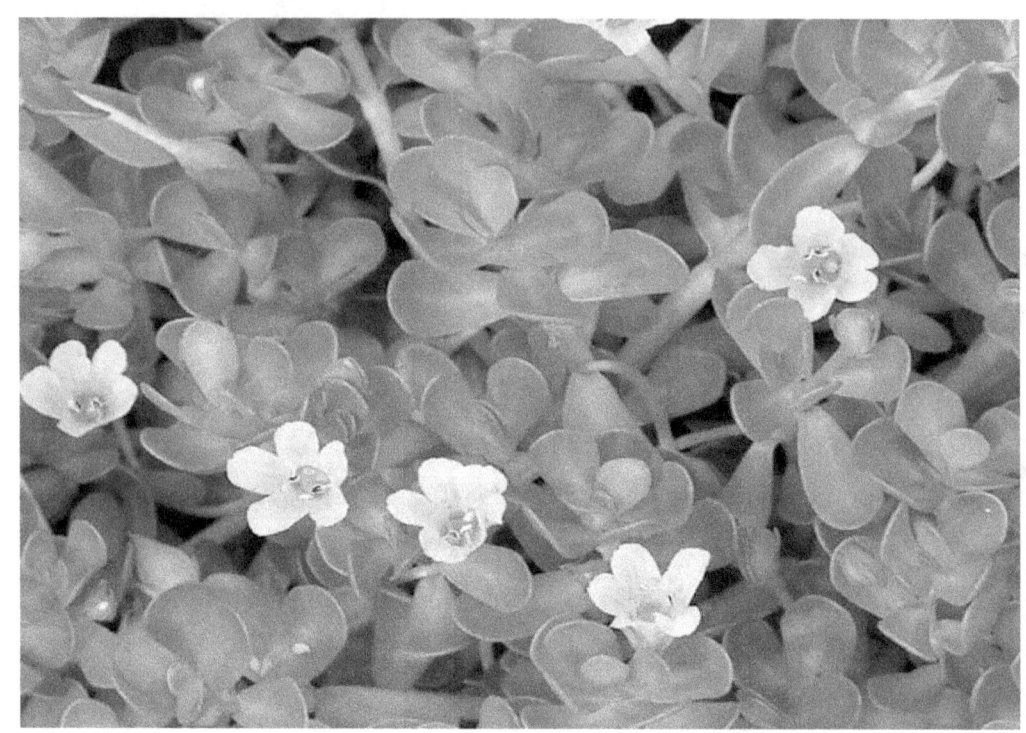

Medicinal properties and uses:-

Brahmi is an ancient and renowned herb considered a significant medicine in Ayurveda. Its properties include enhancing memory, improving mental condition, reducing stress, alleviating sleep problems, and boosting brain performance. It is commonly available in

the form of oil, powder, or capsules, and is typically consumed once or twice a day.

Medicinal properties:-

Brahmi is an ancient herb that offers various health benefits. It has numerous properties, which include the following:-

1. **Memory Enhancement:-** Consuming Brahmi improves memory and recall abilities.

2. **Promoting Stability:-** It helps in enhancing concentration and focus.

3. **Reducing Stress:-** Brahmi can help in alleviating mental stress.

4. **Alleviating Sleep Problems:-** Its consumption aids in achieving better sleep.

5. **Boosting Brain Performance:-** Brahmi increases brain capacity and functionality.

USES:-
Brahmi can be used in several ways:-

1. **For health benefits as an edible food or tea:-** It can be consumed in the form of leaves, or its tea can be made.

2. **As oil or for massage:-** Brahmi oil is available, which can be used for scalp massage.

3. **As an Ayurvedic medicine:-** Brahmi capsules or powder can also be consumed.

4. **For external use:-** It can also be used externally, such as applying it to the skin as a mask or body lotion.

CONCLUSION:-

Brahmi is a powerful herb that can aid in health and development. Its consumption should be well-regulated, and the timing and dosage of all uses should be under the guidance of a medical professional. Before using it, individuals should consult their healthcare specialist.

9. MINT:-

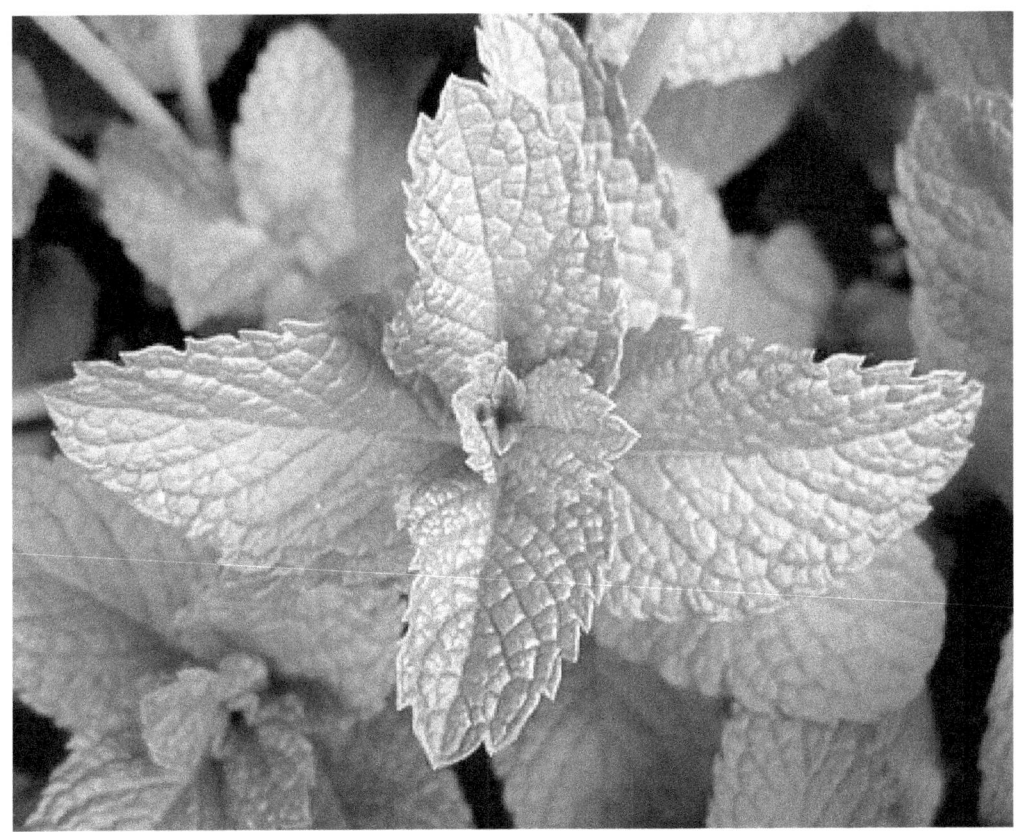

Medicinal properties and uses:-

Mint is a famous and effective herb that helps in enhancing health and freshness. It has many medicinal properties, such as:-

1. **Digestive Power:-** Consuming mint improves digestion and reduces indigestion.

2. **Cooling Effect:-** Its consumption provides physical and mental cooling.

3. **Boosts Immunity:-** Mint contains vitamin C and other antioxidants that enhance the body's immune power.

4. **Revitalizing Properties:-** Its consumption helps alleviate fatigue and anxiety, thereby invigorating the body.

5. **Improves Breathing:-** Consuming mint makes breathing easier and cleanses the lungs.

USES:-

Mint can be used in various forms:-

1. Culinary Use:- Mint chutney, pickles, and mint tea can be made.

2. Medicinal Use:- Directly eating mint leaves or drinking mint tea benefits health.

3. Skincare:- Mint oil is useful for the skin, providing cooling effects and reducing itching.

4. Spices:- Mint can be used in spices, enhancing the flavor of food.

CONCLUSION:-

Mint is a powerful medicinal herb that can help enhance health and freshness. It can be consumed in various forms such as culinary use, medicinal applications, and skincare. It is a common and safe plant suitable for most people.

10. <u>ASHWAGANDHA</u>:-

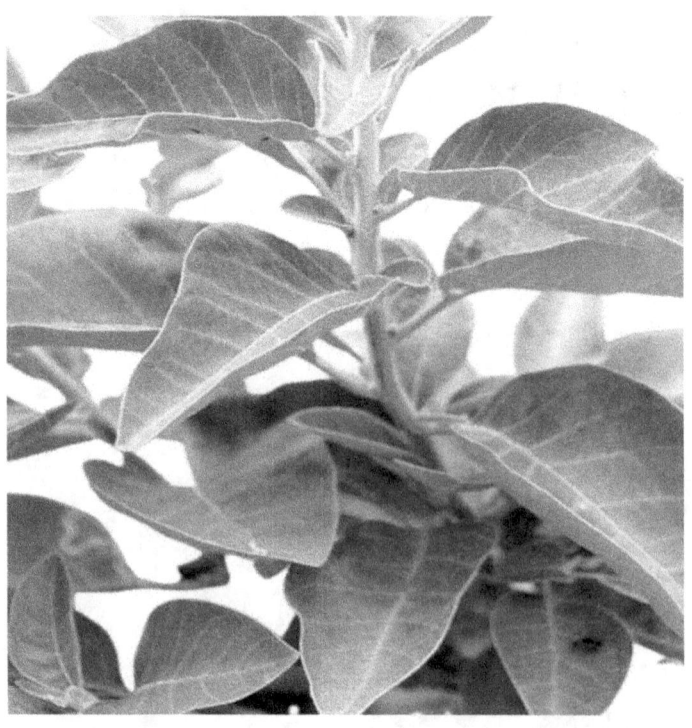

Medicinal properties and uses:-

Ashwagandha, which is also known as "Ashwagandha" in Hindi, is an ancient and renowned herb that holds a significant place in Ayurvedic medicine. Its medicinal properties offer various benefits, such as:-

1. Reducing stress:- Ashwagandha helps in reducing stress and boosts self-confidence.

2. Boosting energy:- It provides the body with energy and freshness, reducing the feeling of fatigue.

3. Enhancing immunity:- Ashwagandha strengthens the immune system, increasing the body's resistance.

4. Coping with heavy medications:- It helps the body cope with heavy medications and strengthens it.

5. Improving focus and perception:- Due to its properties, Ashwagandha improves mental peace and focus.

USES:-

Ashwagandha can be used in various forms:-

1. Powder or capsules:- It is available in powder or capsule form, which can be taken to reap health benefits.

2. Oil or lotion:- Ashwagandha oil or lotion is useful for skin purification.

3. Decoction or tea:- Consuming Ashwagandha in the form of a decoction or tea promotes health and helps in reducing stress.

CONCLUSION:-

Ashwagandha is a major medicinal herb that can help enhance health and vitality. It can be used in various forms, such as powder, capsules, oil, and tea. It is a safe and natural remedy that can aid in improving physical and mental health.

11. **ALOE VERA:-**

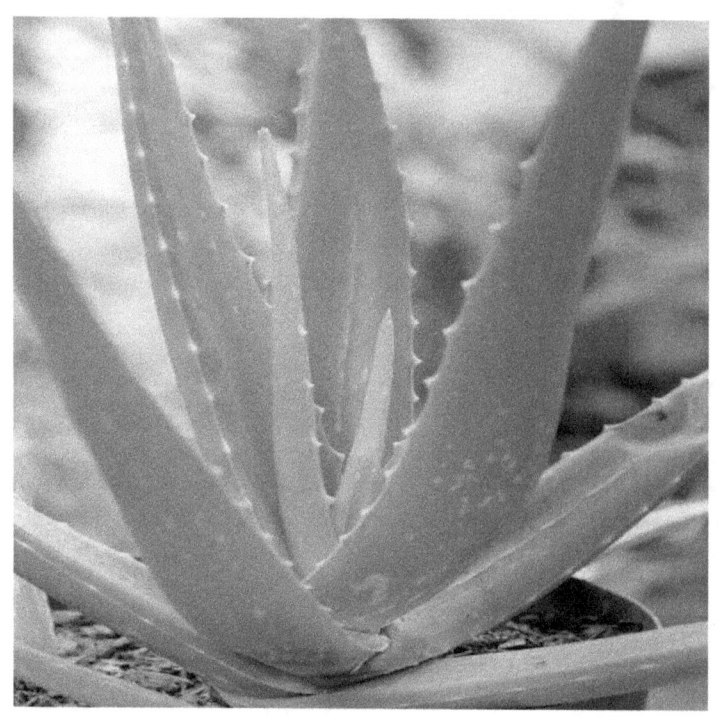

Medicinal properties and uses:-

Aloe Vera is an extremely beneficial herb that aids in the treatment of various health problems. Its main medicinal properties are as follows:-

1. Skin Care:- The most prominent property of Aloe Vera is its use in skin care. It is useful for treating burns, cuts, scrapes, and sunburn.

2. Treatment of Skin Disorders:- Aloe Vera has anti-inflammatory and antiseptic properties that help in treating eczema, psoriasis, and other skin infections.

3. Digestive Health:- Aloe Vera juice helps in improving the digestive system. It aids in relieving constipation, acidity, and other stomach issues.

4. Immunity Booster:- The vitamins and minerals present in Aloe Vera help in strengthening the immune system.

5. Hair Care:- Aloe Vera gel nourishes the scalp and helps in reducing dandruff and hair fall.

6. Antioxidant Properties:- It has antioxidant properties that help in destroying free radicals in the body, protecting cells from damage.

USES:-

Aloe Vera can be used in various ways:-

1. Topical Application:- Applying Aloe Vera gel directly to the skin relieves burns, cuts, and sunburns. It moisturizes the skin and makes it soft.

2. Hair Application:- Apply Aloe Vera gel to the hair and leave it for 30 minutes before washing. This strengthens the hair and keeps the scalp healthy.

3. Aloe Vera Juice:- Drinking Aloe Vera juice regularly strengthens the digestive system and boosts energy levels in the body.

4. Supplements:- Aloe Vera capsules and tablets are available in the market and are used to promote health.

5. Beauty Products:- Aloe Vera is used in many beauty products such as face creams, lotions, shampoos, and conditioners.

CONCLUSION:-

Aloe Vera is a versatile herb that plays a significant role in both health and beauty. Its medicinal properties are highly beneficial for the skin, hair, and digestive system. Regular use of Aloe Vera keeps the skin healthy and radiant, strengthens the hair, and maintains a healthy digestive system. Aloe Vera is a natural and safe remedy that promotes both health and beauty.

12. **GINGER**:-

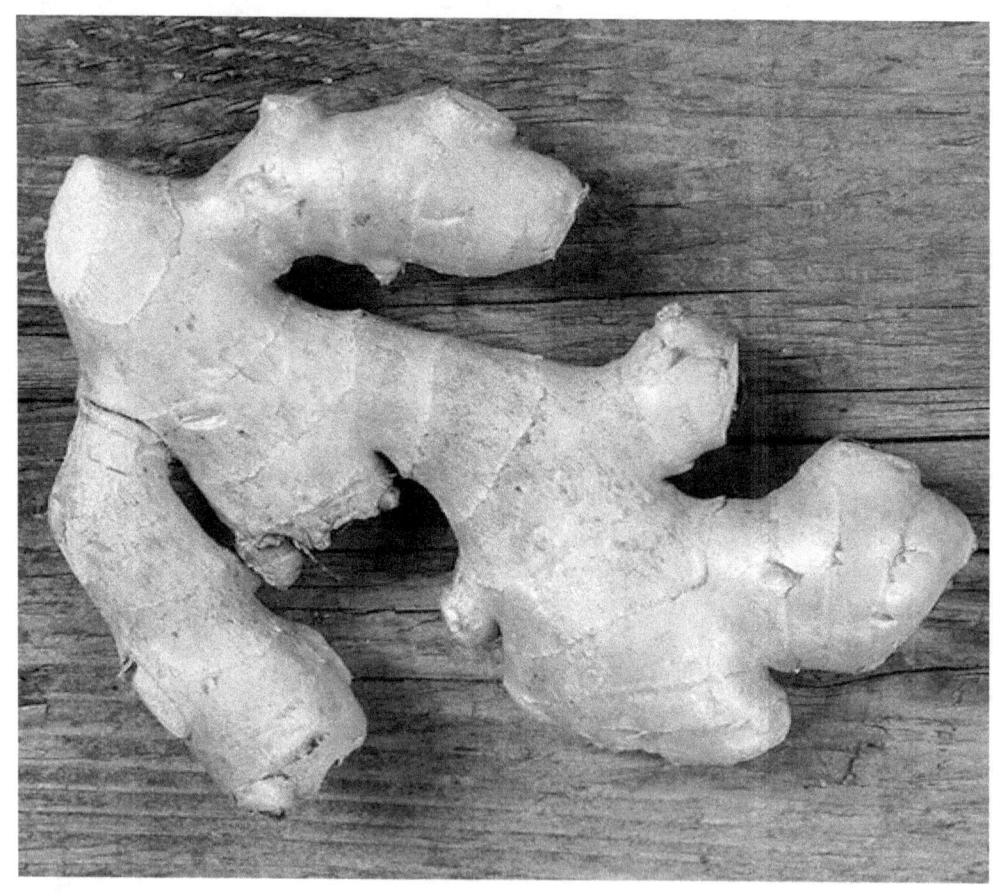

Medicinal properties and uses:-

Ginger is a renowned and widely used herb known for its medicinal properties. Its major medicinal properties are as follows:-

1. Improving Digestion:- Ginger helps in improving the digestive system. It alleviates problems like indigestion, gas, and bloating.

2. Anti-inflammatory:- Ginger has anti-inflammatory properties that help reduce inflammation and pain.

3. Boosting Immunity:- Ginger contains antioxidants that boost the body's immune system and help fight infections.

4. Preventing Nausea and Vomiting:- Consuming ginger is effective in preventing nausea and vomiting in pregnant women.

5. Respiratory Health:- Consuming ginger helps in alleviating issues like colds, coughs, and sore throats.

6. Blood Sugar Control:- Consuming ginger can help in controlling blood sugar levels.

7. Heart Health:- Regular consumption of ginger improves heart health and helps in controlling blood pressure.

USES:-

Ginger can be used in various forms:-

1. As tea:- Ginger tea is beneficial for relieving digestion issues and colds.

2. As a spice in food:- Ginger is used as a spice in various dishes, enhancing the flavor of the food and improving digestion.

3. In juice or soup:- Consuming ginger in juice or soup provides health benefits.

4. For arthritis and muscle pain:- Applying ginger oil or paste to the affected area helps reduce inflammation and pain.

5. To strengthen the immune system:- Ginger can be consumed with honey and lemon, which helps in strengthening the immune system.

CONCLUSION:-

Ginger is a versatile and medicinal herb that is beneficial for various aspects of health. Its medicinal properties help improve digestion, reduce inflammation, boost immunity, and enhance respiratory health. Ginger can be used in various forms, such as tea, spice, juice, and oil. Regular consumption of ginger promotes health and helps prevent various illnesses. Ginger is a natural and safe remedy that is easily available and widely useful.

13. **LEMON**:-

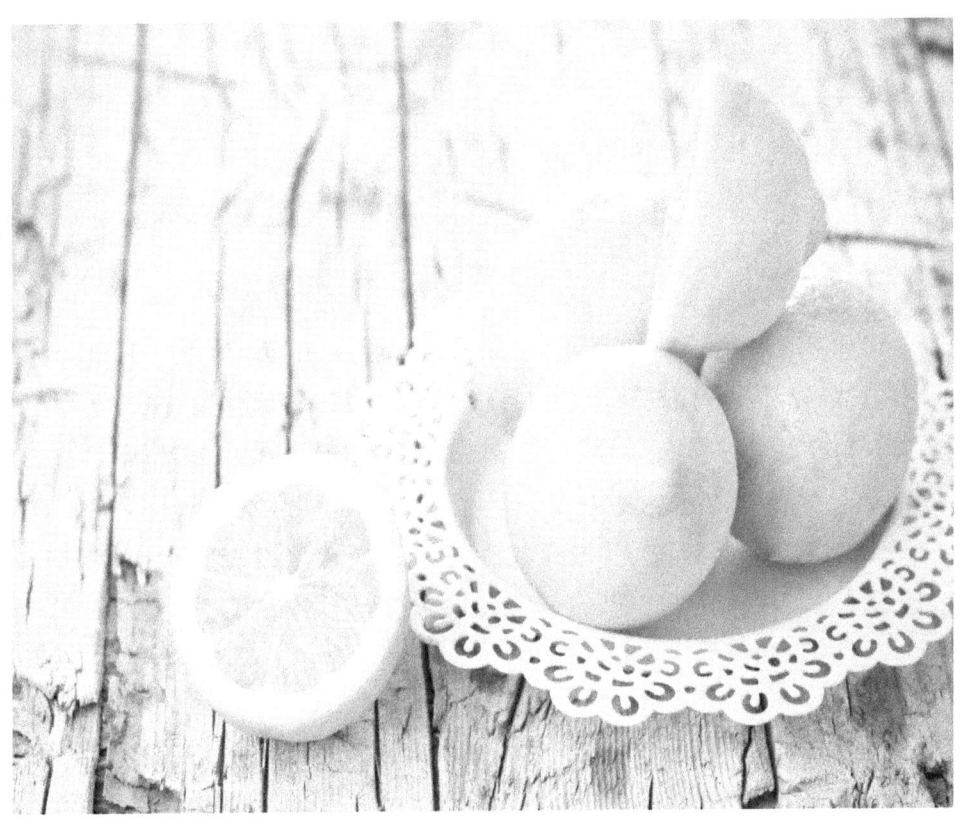

Medicinal properties and uses:-

1. Lemon is a good source of Vitamin C, which helps strengthen the immune system.

2. It contains antioxidants that promote health by destroying body toxins.

3. Lemon juice contains potassium, which improves heart health and reduces the risk of heart diseases.

USAGE:-

1. Mixing lemon juice in cold water during summer helps reduce body heat.

2. Lemon juice removes bad breath and helps in addressing oral problems.

3. Lemon juice enhances hair shine and helps make dry hair soft and healthy.

CONCLUSION:-

Lemon is a beneficial fruit that is a good source of Vitamin C, antioxidants, potassium, and other nutrients. Its use helps improve health, balance digestion, and fight infections.

14. **FENUGREEK**:-

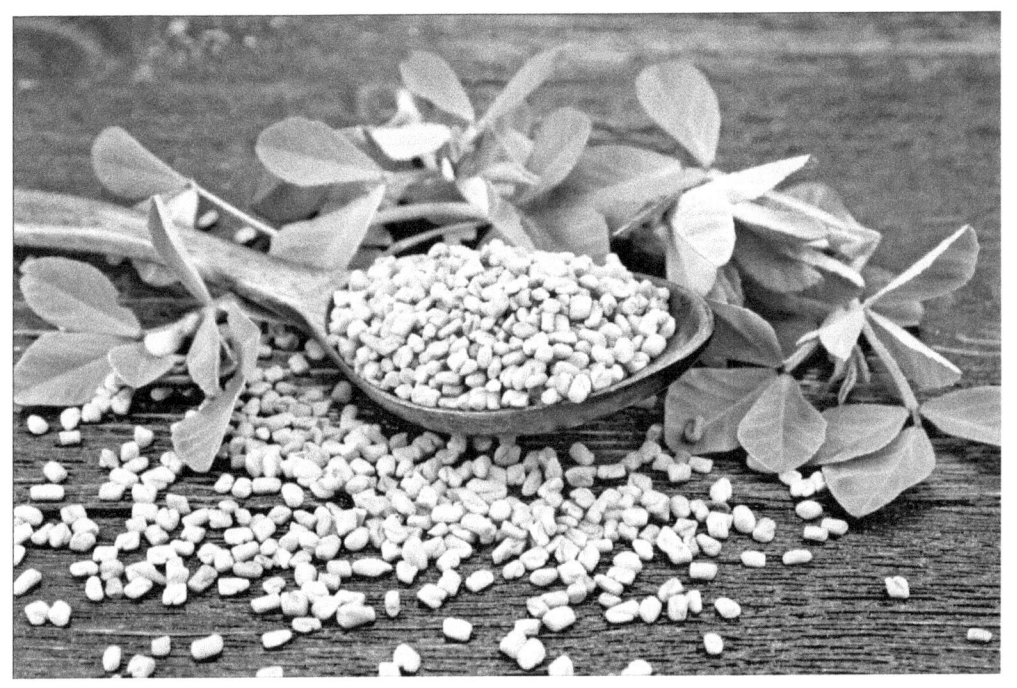

Medicinal properties and uses:-

Fenugreek is an important medicinal plant with numerous health benefits. Some of its key medicinal properties are as follows

1. Blood Sugar Control:- Fenugreek seeds contain soluble fiber called galactomannan, which helps control blood sugar levels.

2. **Improving Digestion:-** Fenugreek seeds aid in digestion and reduce problems such as constipation, bloating, and indigestion.

3. **Lowering Cholesterol:-** Regular consumption of fenugreek seeds helps lower cholesterol levels.

4. **Anti-inflammatory Properties:-** Fenugreek has anti-inflammatory properties that help reduce inflammation and pain.

5. **Increasing Milk Production:-** Fenugreek helps increase milk production for breastfeeding mothers.

6. **Antioxidant Properties:-** The antioxidants present in fenugreek seeds protect the body from free radicals.

USAGE:-

Fenugreek can be used in various ways, as follows:-

1. **In Food:-** Fenugreek leaves and seeds are used in various dishes. They are added to vegetables, lentils, and breads to enhance flavor and nutrition.

2. **Soaked in Water:-** Soaking fenugreek seeds in water overnight and consuming them on an empty stomach in the morning has positive effects on digestion and blood sugar.

3. **As Tea:-** Drinking fenugreek tea improves health and provides relief from colds and coughs.

4. **In Oil and Massage:-** Using fenugreek seeds in sesame oil or other oils for massage benefits the skin and hair.

5. **As Powder:-** Grinding fenugreek seeds into a powder and consuming it provides relief from various health issues.

CONCLUSION:-

The medicinal properties of fenugreek make it an important natural remedy. Regular use can benefit various health issues. Including fenugreek in our daily diet can help maintain health. Considering its benefits, it is not wrong to say that fenugreek is a valuable and versatile medicinal plant.

15. AJWAIN:-

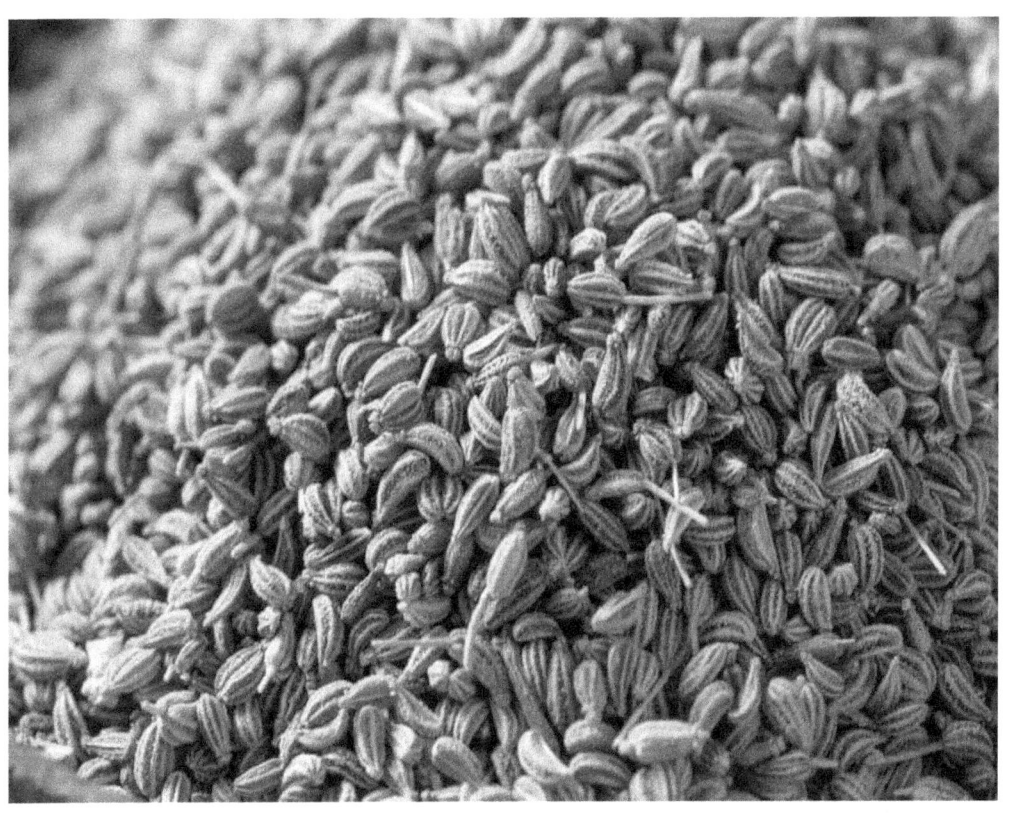

Medicinal properties and uses:-

1. Improving Digestion:- The thymol and other essential oils found in carom seeds activate and strengthen the digestive system. They help reduce gas, indigestion, and stomach pain.

2. Antibacterial and Antifungal Properties:- Carom seeds have antibacterial and antifungal properties, which help fight infections.

3. Reducing Inflammation:- Consuming carom seeds reduces inflammation, which is beneficial in arthritis and other inflammatory diseases.

4. Controlling Diabetes:- Consuming carom seeds can help control blood sugar levels, benefiting diabetic patients.

5. Regulating Blood Pressure:- The elements found in carom seeds help regulate blood pressure, reducing the risk of heart-related problems.

USAGE:-

1. For Digestive Problems:- Chewing roasted or raw carom seeds helps relieve digestive problems. They can be taken with lukewarm water.

2. For Cold and Cough:- Boiling carom seeds in hot water to make a decoction provides relief from cold and cough.

3. For Joint Pain:- Massaging with carom seed oil helps reduce pain and inflammation in the joints.

4. For Diabetes:- Drinking carom seed water on an empty stomach daily can improve blood sugar levels.

5. For Regulating Blood Pressure:- Regular consumption of carom seeds helps regulate blood pressure.

CONCLUSION:-

The medicinal properties and uses of carom seeds are highly effective. Regular and proper consumption can provide benefits for digestive problems, infections, inflammation, diabetes, and blood pressure. Known as an important spice in Indian kitchens, carom seeds not only enhance the flavor of food but are also extremely beneficial for health. Utilizing their natural properties can help us improve our health.

www.ingramcontent.com/pod-product-compliance
Lightning Source LLC
Chambersburg PA
CBHW072000210526
45479CB00003B/1013